Thyroid Connection Cookbook

50 Thyroid Support Meals

Bolster Thyroid Function With a Well-Balanced Diet

By: Timothy Warren

legal or professional, a practiced individual in the profession should be ordered.

Table of Contents

Introduction

Are you looking for recipes that are actually good for your thyroid? Well then, this is definitely the cookbook you are looking for!

This book contains no-nonsense dietary guidelines to treat or prevent thyroid conditions, especially hyperthyroidism and hypothyroidism. Best of all, this is a cookbook filled with a wide variety of delicious, nutritious and easy-to-prepare recipes that will help to not just support healthy thyroid function but also improve your overall physical and mental well-being. You will find recipes for breakfast, snacks, soups, stews, vegetable and meat-based main dishes and even whole grains and desserts.

If you are someone who has just been diagnosed with a thyroid condition, or if you are at risk of developing one, then you will definitely need this book in your life. Just make sure to discuss everything with your doctor before you get into any sort of treatment and dietary program. This book is also for those who are healthy are looking for even more delicious recipes to prepare at home.

So show your body some love and start making your own healthy thyroid support meals now!

Chapter 1 – Dietary Guidelines for a Healthy Thyroid

Hello there! You might be reading this book because you have a thyroid condition, or that you are concerned about the health of your thyroid gland. Well, we'll definitely get into the dietary guidelines for that, but first let's talk a little bit more about the thyroid.

Get to Know the Thyroid

The thyroid is a ductless, butterfly-shaped gland found close to the base of the neck. It is responsible for releasing the hormones that regulate your metabolism. Thus, it has a direct effect on all your body's main functions, including your body temperature, heart rate, breathing, cholesterol levels, and so on.

The two main hormones it produces are called *triiodothyronine* (T3) and *thyroxine* (T4). It is crucial for the levels of these two hormones to remain stable, and so, to maintain this balance, the hypothalamus and pituitary glands (found in the brain) work together.

Specifically, the hypothalamus excretes the TSH Releasing Hormone that triggers the pituitary gland to send a signal to the thyroid gland to produce specific levels of T3 and T4.

However, if there is miscommunication between any of these three important glands, the T3 and T4 levels become too high or too low.

If they are too low in the blood, the result is a slower than normal heart rate and weight gain. The person would also be constantly experiencing constipation. This condition is known as **hypothyroidism**. People who suffer from this condition also tend to experience symptoms such as lack of focus, insomnia, lethargy, muscular and joint pain, and heavy, frequent periods.

On the other hand, if they are too high, the person would suffer from **hyperthyroidism.** The symptoms are usually a combination of a rapid heart rate and extreme weight loss. He or she would also constantly suffer from diarrhea. Hair loss, light or missed menstrual periods, anxiety and hyperactivity are also known symptoms of this condition.

As you can see, it is important to develop the right habits in order to maintain a healthy thyroid gland. To help treat your thyroid condition or maintain proper thyroid function, you should nourish your body with the right nutrients and avoid foods that might negatively affect this delicate balance.

The Dietary Guidelines

Depending on your thyroid condition, certain foods should be eaten in moderation as they can negatively impact your medication or treatment. However, there are also foods that should be avoided altogether. Carefully read the following guidelines and seek to implement them into your dietary lifestyle:

1. Avoid Fatty Food

   Fats are scientifically proven to reduce the effectiveness of thyroid hormone replacement medication. Furthermore, they may have a direct impact on the thyroid's functions. On top of that, saturated fats and hydrogenated oils are just downright bad for your health. So, try your best to reduce the amount of animal fat, butter, margarine, and anything with the word" hydrogenated" from your diet, and avoid deep-fried foods at all costs.

2. Reduce Sugar Intake

   Processed sugar is all calories and zero nutrients, which is bad news to not just those who have an existing thyroid condition but also anyone who wants to stay fit and healthy. To add some sweetness to your dishes, always choose all-natural, organic sources, such as raw honey and maple syrup, because they have added benefits besides the flavor. However, it is still best to enjoy them in limited portions.

3. Eat less cruciferous vegetables if you have hypothyroidism, more if you have hyperthyroidism

   People who have hypothyroidism, especially if they have iodine deficiency should reduce the amount of cruciferous vegetables in their diet. This is because food like cauliflower, broccoli, Brussels sprouts, cabbage, and bok choy contain phytochemicals that can prevent the thyroid from absorbing the iodine it needs to function properly. You can still enjoy these foods (as they are both scrumptious and extremely nutritious) as long as you cook them and limit your portions to at most 5 ounces per day.

   If you have hyperthyroidism, however, you are free to eat as much cruciferous vegetables as you like, since they do naturally reduce the thyroid function. You can even reduce the amount of antithyroid medication by eating cruciferous

4. Eliminate soy if you have hypothyroidism, consider consuming more if you have hyperthyroidism

   Soy is high in *phytoestrogen*, which inhibits the absorption of the thyroid hormone. While more research is needed to identify its direct affects to hypothyroidism, it is best to be safe by limiting your portions of this food.

   On the other hand, if you have hyperthyroidism you should consult your doctor about consuming more soy first before you try anything.

5. Eliminate gluten *if* you are sensitive or intolerant to it

   Whole grains are an important part of a healthy, well-balanced diet. However, if you are taking thyroid hormone replacement medication, you should talk to your doctor about reducing the amount of gluten you consume. This is because some people are gluten sensitive, meaning they cannot absorb much of the nutrients from their food if the gluten irritates their small intestine.

6. If you drink coffee, do so only *after* taking thyroid medication.

Coffee has a direct impact against your body's ability to absorb your thyroid replacement medication, so make sure to enjoy it only after at least an hour of taking your pill.

7. Enjoy fiber-rich food in moderation.

   Fiber is an integral component in a healthy diet. It helps cleanse the digestive tract so that you can absorb the nutrients from your food better. It is also necessary to help relieve you of constipation. However, when you have hypothyroidism, it might cause complications to your medication. Ask your doctor about the right amount of grams of fiber per day for you, then adjust your portions accordingly.

8. Eliminate processed food and choose whole food whenever possible.

   The problem with processed food is that you are not sure of what's inside them, and uncertainty is the last thing you want if you have a thyroid condition. Processed food is especially high in fat, sodium, and sugar, three of the worst ingredients to put inside your body.

Avoid them entirely and stick to whole foods, or foods fresh from nature.

9. Avoid alcohol and drink more water.

   Alcohol contributes to the imbalance of the production of the thyroid hormones and in fact causes damaging effects on the thyroid gland itself. It also has dehydrating effects on your body.

   Water, on the other hand, flushes out the toxins from your body and hydrates the cells. It is important for you to stay hydrated, especially if you have a thyroid condition. Aim to drink two glasses of water before and after each meal, and to hydrate whenever you remember to do so.

10. Monitor your iodine intake.

   One of the main reasons why people suffer from hypothyroidism is iodine deficiency. Since iodine is not produced by the body, it is important to consume foods that contain it. However, too much iodine in the blood has also led to the development of autoimmune thyroid disease. This is because iodine inhibits the function of the thyroid peroxidase, an enzyme that plays a critical role in the production of the thyroid hormone.

   As someone who has or is at risk of a thyroid condition, it is important for you to monitor the amount of iodine in your blood. You must also talk to your doctor about taking selenium along with your iodine.

All these factors might sound a bit complicated, but in truth it becomes simple once you embrace a healthy, well-balanced diet. If you consume healthy food in moderate portions *and* make sure to remember your doctor's advice (such as minimizing the amount of cruciferous vegetables and soy for those with hypothyroidism), then you will be able to bolster your thyroid function and treat its condition.

The best way to follow a balanced diet and monitor the types of foods you consume is to cook them at home. Plan and make your meals ahead so that you can spend less time and energy cooking. Buy your ingredients in bulk so that you can save a significant amount of money from your food budget. Most importantly, enjoy the process of cooking your own food as much as you like eating them. Your thyroid – and your health in general, for that matter – will simply reflect the healthy new lifestyle you have adapted.

Now, you can go right ahead and start whipping up your own healthy, thyroid-friendly meals.

Chapter 2 – Breakfast

Cinnamon Cocoa French Toast

Number of Servings: 3

You will need:

- 6 slices whole wheat or gluten-free bread
- 1 banana, peeled and sliced thinly
- 4 strawberries, sliced thinly
- ½ cup water
- 1/3 cup chopped cashews
- ¾ Tbsp cacao powder
- ¾ tsp whole wheat flour
- 1/3 tsp pure vanilla extract
- 1/3 tsp ground cinnamon
- Nonstick cooking spray

How to Prepare:

1. Soak the cashews in water for about 3 hours, then drain and rinse well.

2. Pour the cashews into a food processor and add the water, cacao powder, flour, vanilla extract, and cinnamon. Blend until smooth.

3. Coat the skillet with nonstick cooking spray, then heat over medium high flame.

4. Dip the slices of bread into the flour mixture, then cook in the skillet for 4 minutes per side, or until lightly crisp and brown.

5. Transfer the French toast to a plate and top with sliced banana and strawberries. Serve right away.

Easy Buckwheat Pancakes

Number of Servings: 4

You will need:

- 1 large egg white
- 1 cup skim milk
- ¾ cup whole wheat flour
- 1/3 cup buckwheat flour
- 2 ½ Tbsp unsweetened apple juice concentrate
- 1 tsp low sodium baking powder

How to Prepare:

1. Sift the whole wheat and buckwheat flours and baking powder into a bowl, then set aside.
2. In a separate bowl, beat the egg white with the skim milk and apple juice concentrate. Gradually stir the egg white mixture into the flour mixture until just combined. A few lumps are fine.
3. Place a pancake griddle over medium flame and heat through. If needed, add a bit of nonstick cooking spray.

4. Ladle a quarter cup of the batter on the hot griddle and cook for 2 minutes per side, or until firm.

5. Stack the pancakes on a platter and serve right away with fresh fruit.

Banana Oat Bran Bowls

Number of Servings: 2

You will need:

- 3 large bananas, peeled
- 1 ½ cups unsweetened almond milk
- ¾ cup organic oat bran
- 2 Tbsp ground flaxseeds
- 2 tsp raw honey
- ½ tsp ground cinnamon

How to Prepare:

1. Combine all the ingredients and two of the bananas in a blender. Blend until smooth.
2. Divide between two bowls. Slice the bananas thinly, then divide between two servings. Serve right away.

Cinnamon Raisin Oatmeal

Number of Servings: 3

You will need:

- 1 ½ cups water
- ¾ cup sweetened almond milk
- ¾ cup traditional rolled oats
- 1/3 cup raisins
- ¾ tsp ground cinnamon
- Sea salt, to taste

How to Prepare:

1. Pour the water into a saucepan, then place over medium high flame and bring to a boil. Once boiling, stir in the oats, then reduce to low flame and simmer for 10 minutes, or until thickened.
2. Stir in the raisins and simmer for 5 minutes, stirring occasionally.
3. Turn off the heat, then stir in the ground cinnamon and a dash of sea salt. Mix well, then stir in the milk until combined.

4. Ladle into bowls and serve right away.

Chai Pumpkin Waffles

Number of Servings: 6

You will need:

- 3 ½ cups milk
- 1 ½ cups whole wheat flour
- 1 ½ cups all-purpose flour
- 1 cup pureed pumpkin
- 4 Tbsp flaxseed meal
- 4 tsp baking powder
- 2 tsp pure vanilla extract
- 2 tsp apple cider vinegar
- 1 tsp sea salt
- 1 tsp powdered stevia
- 1 tsp ground cinnamon
- ½ tsp baking soda
- ½ tsp allspice
- ½ tsp ground cardamom
- Freshly ground black pepper, to taste

- Nonstick cooking spray

How to Prepare:

1. Combine the all-purpose flour and whole wheat flour with the flaxseed meal, salt, baking soda, baking powder, ground cinnamon, allspice, cardamom, and powdered stevia. Stir in a pinch of black pepper and set aside.
2. In a bowl, combine the apple cider vinegar with the milk. Stir in the vanilla extract, then fold in the pureed pumpkin. Mix well until smooth.
3. Stir the flour mixture into the pumpkin mixture, then set aside for 15 minutes.
4. Meanwhile, coat the waffle iron with nonstick cooking spray. Pour in the batter and cook based on waffle iron manufacturer's instructions.
5. Once cooked, transfer the waffles to a plate and serve warm.

Blueberry Quinoa Porridge

Number of Servings: 3

You will need:

- 1 ½ cups water
- 1 ½ cups fresh blueberries (or any other berry in season)
- 1 cup skim, soy, or almond milk
- ¾ cup quinoa
- 2 ½ Tbsp chopped walnuts
- Ground cinnamon, to taste

How to Prepare:

1. Pour the quinoa into a fine mesh strainer, then rinse under cold running water thoroughly. Transfer to a saucepan.
2. Pour the water into the saucepan with the quinoa, then add a pinch of cinnamon. Place over medium high flame and bring to a boil.
3. Once boiling, stir in the walnuts and reduce to low flame. Cover and simmer

for 12 minutes, or until the quinoa has completely absorbed the water.

4. Fluff up the quinoa, then stir in the milk. Fold in the blueberries, then serve right away.

Chapter 3 – Snacks and Smoothies

Pineapple Ginger Smoothie

Number of Servings: 2

You will need:

- 2 frozen pineapples, peeled and chopped
- 4 Tbsp freshly squeezed lemon juice
- 1 inch ginger, peeled
- 2 Tbsp raw honey

How to Prepare:

1. Combine all ingredients into a high power blender. Blend until smooth, then pour into two glasses and serve right away.

Roasted Red Pepper and Garlic Hummus

Number of Servings: 4

You will need:

- 1 large garlic clove, roasted
- 1 cup cooked unsalted, non-fat garbanzo beans, drained thoroughly
- ¼ cup chopped roasted red bell peppers
- 2 ½ Tbsp freshly squeezed lemon juice
- 2 ½ Tbsp tahini
- Dried basil, to taste
- Freshly ground black pepper, to taste

How to Prepare:

2. Pour the garbanzo beans into a food processor, then add the roasted garlic and bell peppers, followed by the lemon juice and tahini.
3. Blend until smooth, then add a pinch of basil and black pepper and blend again. Adjust seasoning to taste, if needed.

4. Pour the hummus into a bowl, cover, and refrigerate until ready to serve.
5. Best served chilled with whole wheat toast or carrot, celery, and cucumber sticks.

Berry Banana Smoothie

Number of Servings: 2

You will need:

- 1 cup raspberries, rinsed and drained thoroughly
- 1 cup blueberries, rinsed and drained thoroughly
- 1 cup sliced strawberries
- ½ cup pomegranate seeds
- 2 frozen bananas, chopped
- 1 Tbsp raw honey

How to Prepare:

1. Combine all ingredients into a high power blender. Blend until smooth, then pour into two glasses and serve right away.

Cheesy Minty Grilled Tomatoes

Number of Servings: 9

You will need:

- 36 cherry tomatoes
- 3 Tbsp freshly shaved Parmesan cheese
- 1 ½ Tbsp pure olive oil
- 1 ½ Tbsp apple cider vinegar
- 1 ½ Tbsp chopped fresh mint
- 1/3 tsp sea salt
- Freshly ground black pepper, to taste

How to Prepare:

2. Preheat the grill to medium heat.
3. Line a rimmed baking sheet aluminum foil, then set aside.
4. Lightly pierce each cherry tomato with a sharp knife, then arrange on them on the prepared baking sheet. Set aside.
5. Mix together the olive oil with the vinegar, then season with salt and a pinch of black pepper.

6. Pour the dressing over the cherry tomatoes, then toss well to coat. Cover the baking sheet with another sheet of aluminum foil, then crimp the edges to seal.

7. Roast the tomatoes for 6 minutes, then carefully place on a cooling sheet. Carefully remove the top sheet of aluminum foil, then transfer to a serving bowl.

8. Stir in the Parmesan cheese and mint, then serve right away.

Minty Spinach and Peach Smoothie

Number of Servings: 2

You will need:

- 2 cups chopped fresh baby spinach, rinsed and drained thoroughly
- 3 peaches, peeled and cored
- 1 large cucumber, peeled
- 6 fresh mint sprigs, rinsed thoroughly
- 2 apples, peeled, cored, and chopped
- 2 Tbsp freshly squeezed lemon juice
- 2 tsp raw honey

How to Prepare:

1. Combine all ingredients into a high power blender. Blend until smooth, then pour into two glasses and serve right away.

Savory Salmon-Stuffed Eggs

Number of Servings: 6

You will need:

- 6 large hard-boiled eggs
- 1 cup chopped fresh curly parsley
- 2 oz boneless cold-smoked salmon
- 1 ½ oz light cream cheese, softened
- 2 Tbsp olive oil mayonnaise
- 1 Tbsp chopped fresh chives
- Freshly ground black pepper, to taste

How to Prepare:

2. Lay the parsley on a serving plate and set aside.
3. Slice the eggs in half, then scoop out the yolks and discard. Arrange the egg whites on top of the parsley and set aside.
4. Place the salmon into a food processor, then add the cream cheese and olive oil mayonnaise. Blend well until smooth, then season to taste with black pepper and blend again.

5. Pour the mixture into a bowl and fold in the chopped fresh chives. Spoon the salmon mixture into the egg whites, then cover the plate and refrigerate until ready to serve.

6. Best served chilled.

Chapter 4 – Soups and Stews

Vegetable Stew for Hyperthyroidism

Number of Servings: 6

You will need:

- 1 ½ Tbsp pure olive oil
- 1 large onion, chopped
- 2 large garlic cloves, crushed
- 2 inches fresh ginger, crushed
- 6 green beans, chopped
- 3 potatoes, peeled and cubed
- 3 carrots, peeled and cubed
- 3 cups chopped cauliflower florets
- 3 cups chopped broccoli florets
- 2 cups shredded green cabbage
- 6 cups water
- 1 tsp raw honey

- ¾ tsp low sodium soy sauce
- 1/3 tsp red chili pepper
- Sea salt

How to Prepare:

1. Place a large saucepan over medium flame and heat the olive oil. Sauté the garlic and ginger until fragrant, then add all the vegetables except the onion and potatoes.

2. Sauté for 5 minutes, or until crisp tender, then add the water and increase heat to high. Once boiling, add the potatoes, chili pepper, and soy sauce. Simmer until tender.

3. Add the honey and onion, then season to taste with sea salt. Simmer for 3 minutes, then ladle into bowls and serve right away.

Ginger and Pumpkin Soup

Number of Servings: 3

You will need:

- 1 small sweet onion, chopped
- 2 carrots, peeled and sliced
- 1 celery stalk, chopped
- 2 cups water
- 1 cup cubed pumpkin
- 1 ½ Tbsp minced fresh ginger
- ¾ Tbsp canola oil
- ¼ tsp ground cinnamon
- 1 bay leaf
- Dried thyme, to taste
- Dried oregano, to taste
- Freshly ground black pepper, to taste

How to Prepare:

1. Place a stock pot over medium flame and heat through. Once hot, add the canola oil and swirl to coat.

2. Sauté the onion and celery until tender, then stir in the carrot, pumpkin, ginger, and bay leaf.

3. Add a pinch of thyme and oregano, then pour in the water and increase to high flame. Bring to a boil, then reduce to medium low flame and cover. Simmer for 20 minutes, tor until the pumpkin and carrot are tender.

4. Discard the bay leaf, then turn off the heat. Mash the solids with a potato masher or an immersion blender.

5. Reheat over low flame, then season to taste with black pepper. Ladle into soup bowls and serve right away.

Indian Tomato Soup

Number of Servings: 3

You will need:

- 8 tomatoes, seeded and chopped
- 1 large garlic clove, crushed
- 1 green chili pepper, seeded and diced
- 3 cups water
- 3 tsp crushed fresh ginger
- ½ Tbsp chopped fresh coriander
- 3 tsp olive oil
- 2 tsp sea salt
- 1 tsp curry powder
- ½ tsp cumin
- ½ tsp freshly ground black pepper
- ¼ tsp black mustard seeds

How to Prepare:

1. Place the tomatoes and garlic into a food processor and blend until pureed. Set aside.

2. Boil the water in a saucepan, then stir in the pureed tomatoes. Add the green chili, coriander, and ginger. Reduce to low flame and simmer for about 3 minutes.

3. Stir in the curry, cumin, salt, and pepper, then simmer for 3 minutes.

4. Meanwhile, heat the olive oil in a saucepan, then stir in the mustard seeds. Reduce to low flame and cover, then cook for 1 minute or until the seeds have popped.

5. Ladle the soup into bowls, then top with the mustard seeds and serve right away.

Irish Leek and Potato Soup

Number of Servings: 3

You will need:

- 1 Tbsp pure olive oil
- 1 small onion, chopped
- 1 leek, chopped
- 3 Yukon Gold potatoes, cubed
- 1 ½ cups chicken broth, unsalted or low sodium
- ½ cup water
- ¾ cup skim milk
- ¼ cup minced fresh chives
- 2 Tbsp chopped fresh parsley
- 1 Tbsp whole wheat flour
- Cayenne pepper, to taste
- Ground nutmeg, to taste

How to Prepare:

1. Place a soup pot over medium flame and heat through. Once hot, add the olive oil and swirl to coat.

2. Sauté the onion and leeks for 5 minutes, then stir in the flour and sauté until simmering.

3. Pour in the water and broth, then add the potatoes. Increase to medium high flame and let simmer, then reduce to low flame and cover. Cook for 15 minutes, or until the potatoes are extra tender.

4. Turn off the heat and mash the potatoes until chunky smooth. Reheat over low flame and stir to combine.

5. Add the milk and stir well, then season with cayenne and nutmeg to taste. Turn off the heat, then stir in the parsley and chives. Serve right away.

Moroccan Carrot Soup

Number of Servings: 6

You will need:

- 6 cups vegetable or chicken broth, unsalted or low sodium
- 6 cups peeled and diced carrot
- 1 ½ lemons
- 2 small garlic cloves, crushed
- 1 ½ Tbsp chopped fresh parsley
- ¾ tsp cayenne pepper
- ¾ tsp paprika
- ¾ tsp raw honey
- 1/3 tsp cumin
- 1/6 tsp ground cinnamon

How to Prepare:

1. Boil the broth in a saucepan, then place the carrots and garlic. Reduce to a simmer, cover, and cook until tender.

2. Turn off the heat and allow to cool slightly. Ladle half the mixture into a food processor and blend until smooth.
3. Stir back into the saucepan and place over low flame. Stir in the cumin, cayenne, cinnamon, and paprika. Simmer until fragrant, then stir and remove from heat.
4. Add the honey and squeeze in the lemon juice. Mix well, then ladle into soup bowls, top with parsley, and serve right away.

Beef and Veggie Stew

Number of Servings: 3

You will need:

- ½ lb stewing beef cubes, fat trimmed off
- 1 small potato, peeled and diced
- 2 turnips, diced
- 2 small tomatoes, chopped
- 3 garlic cloves, minced
- 2 cups beef broth, unsalted or low sodium
- 1 cup diced zucchini
- 1/3 cup diced onion
- ¼ cup diced celery
- ¼ cup diced carrot
- 2 Tbsp whole wheat flour
- 1 Tbsp pure olive oil
- 1 Tbsp Worcestershire sauce
- ½ bay leaf
- 2 fresh thyme sprigs

- Freshly ground black pepper, to taste

How to Prepare:

1. Place a stock pot over medium flame and heat through. Once hot, add the olive oil and swirl to coat. Add the beef cubes and cook until browned all over.

2. Scatter the flour over the beef cubes, then stir well to coat. Stir in the onion, celery, garlic, leek, potato, turnip, zucchini, and tomato. Mix well, then pour in the broth and stir in the bay leaf and thyme.

3. Increase flame and bring to a boil. Once boiling, reduce to medium low flame, cover, and cook for 30 to 45 minutes, or until the beef is fork tender.

4. Discard the thyme sprigs and bay leaf, then stir in the Worcestershire sauce. Season to taste with black pepper, then serve piping hot.

Chapter 5 – Vegetable Dishes

Grilled Vegetable Feast

Number of Servings: 4

You will need:

- 1 large red bell pepper, seeded and quartered
- 1 large green bell pepper, seeded and quartered
- 1 large zucchini, halved lengthwise and cut into bite-sized pieces
- 1 medium yellow squash, peeled and cut into bite-sized pieces
- 3 green onions, white and light green parts, chopped
- 2 cups fresh mushrooms, any kind, sliced
- ¾ tsp dried basil
- ¾ tsp dried thyme
- Garlic powder, to taste
- Mustard powder, to taste

- Freshly ground black pepper, to taste
- Nonstick cooking spray

How to Prepare:

1. Preheat the grill to medium flame.
2. Cover a large grill pan with aluminum foil, then lightly coat with nonstick cooking spray.
3. Spread all the vegetables on the roasting pan, then sprinkle with the garlic powder, mustard powder, thyme, basil, and black pepper. Toss lightly to coat.
4. Cover the roasting pan with another sheet of aluminum foil and crimp the edges to seal.
5. Grill the vegetables for 25 minutes, or until all the vegetables are fork tender.
6. Carefully remove the aluminum foil cover from the vegetables, then grill for 5 minutes. Adjust seasoning, if needed.
7. Transfer to a serving platter and serve right away.

Spinach, Sweet Potato and Lentil Curry

Number of Servings: 6

You will need:

- 1 ½ Tbsp pure olive oil
- 1 large onion, chopped
- 3 garlic cloves, crushed
- 2 inches fresh ginger, peeled and minced
- 1 large sweet potato, peeled and cubed
- 5 oz baby spinach
- 2 cups dried lentils, rinsed
- 3 cups vegetable broth, unsalted or low sodium
- 3 Tbsp chopped almonds
- 1 ½ Tbsp curry powder
- 1 ½ tsp ground cumin
- Sea salt, to taste
- Freshly ground black pepper, to taste

How to Prepare:

1. Place a saucepan over medium flame and heat through. Once hot, add the olive oil and sauté the onion until translucent. Add the garlic and sauté until fragrant.
2. Add the curry, cumin, and ginger. Stir well, then add the lentils and broth. Bring to a boil, then reduce to a simmer. Cover and simmer for 10 minutes.
3. After 10 minutes, stir in the sweet potato and cover. Simmer for 10 minutes or until tender.
4. Add the spinach and cook until wilted. Season to taste with salt and pepper.
5. Ladle into soup bowls and top with chopped almonds. Serve right away.

Savory Stewed Greens

Number of Servings: 6

You will need:

- 1 large red onion, minced
- 6 tomatoes, chopped
- 1 green chili pepper, seeded and minced
- 1 small lemon
- 4 cups collard greens, washed and chopped
- 3 cups spinach, rinsed and drained thoroughly
- 3 cups chopped kale
- 1 cup water
- 4 Tbsp pure olive oil
- 1 ½ Tbsp whole wheat flour
- ½ tsp sea salt
- ¼ tsp freshly ground black pepper

How to Prepare:

1. Steam the greens for about 6 minutes or until tender. Transfer to a colander and set aside.

2. Place a large saucepan over medium flame and heat through. Once hot, add 3 tablespoons olive oil and swirl to coat. Sauté the onion, chili pepper, and tomatoes. Simmer for 5 minutes, then reduce to low flame. Add the remaining olive oil.

3. Juice the lemon into a bowl. Stir in half the water and all the flour. Mix well, then pour into the saucepan and stir well to combine.

4. Add all the water into the saucepan, then add the greens and season with salt and pepper. Stir well, then set to medium flame and cover. Cook for 3 minutes, or until tender.

Steamed Asparagus and Sun-Dried Tomatoes

Number of Servings: 4

You will need:

- 15 oz asparagus, trimmed
- 4 Tbsp chopped fresh basil
- 4 Tbsp chopped sun-dried tomatoes
- 2 Tbsp chopped fresh parsley
- 2 Tbsp extra virgin olive oil
- 2 tsp flaxseed oil
- 2 tsp balsamic vinegar
- 1 tsp cayenne pepper

How to Prepare:

1. Combine the extra virgin olive oil with the flaxseed oil, balsamic vinegar, and cayenne pepper in a bowl.
2. Add the sun-dried tomatoes and 1 tablespoon of parsley. Mix well, then cover and set aside for at least 2 hours.
3. Boil water in a steamer, then add the asparagus in the steamer basket. Steam for about 5 minutes, or until fork tender.

4. Lay the steamed asparagus on a serving plate, then drizzle the sauce on top. Toss to coat, then top with basil and parsley. Serve right away.

Spinach and Apple Salad

Number of Servings: 3

You will need:

- 150 grams spinach, chopped
- 5 apples
- 5 spring onions, chopped
- 5 celery stalks, chopped
- 3 lemons
- 6 Tbsp tahini
- 6 Tbsp olive oil mayonnaise
- 6 Tbsp sesame seeds
- 3 Tbsp raw honey

How to Prepare:

1. Combine the celery and onions in a bowl. Core and dice the apples, then add to the celery mixture and toss well.
2. Juice one lemon over everything and toss well to coat. Refrigerate and set aside.
3. Meanwhile, combine the olive oil mayonnaise, honey, and tahini. Juice the

remaining lemons over the mixture, then whisk well to combine.

4. Pour the dressing over the apple mixture, then toss well to coat. Refrigerate for an hour, or until chilled.
5. To serve, spread the spinach on a serving dish and add the apple salad on top. Sprinkle with sesame seeds, then serve right away.

Tunisian Hot Veggie Salad

Number of Servings: 3

You will need:

- 6 tomatoes
- 3 large red bell pepper
- 3 large red onions
- 1 ½ lemons
- 6 Tbsp crumbled feta cheese
- 4 ½ Tbsp olive oil
- 15 oz canned tuna packed in brine, drained thoroughly
- 1 ½ tsp dried oregano
- Sea salt, to taste
- Freshly ground black pepper, to taste

How to Prepare:

1. Set the oven to 400 degrees F to preheat.
2. Poke the peppers and tomatoes with a sharp knife. Place the peppers, tomatoes, and onions on a baking sheet

and roast for about 20 minutes, turning once, until tender and browned.

3. Transfer the roasted veggies to a bowl and set aside to cool slightly. Once cooled, peel the skins off and chop. Lay on a serving dish, then add the tuna and feta cheese on top.

4. Juice the lemon over the salad, then add the olive oil, oregano, salt, and pepper. Toss gently, then serve right away.

Hot Potato and Broccoli Salad

Number of Servings: 6

You will need:

- 4 large potatoes, peeled and cubed
- 2 green onions, white and light green parts, chopped
- 1 large garlic clove, minced
- 1 ½ cups chopped broccoli florets
- 2 ½ Tbsp freshly squeezed lemon juice
- 2 Tbsp pure olive oil
- 2 Tbsp white wine vinegar
- 1 ½ tsp dried parsley
- 1/3 tsp dried basil
- Mustard powder, to taste
- Dijon mustard, to taste
- Dried red pepper flakes, to taste

How to Prepare:

1. Set the oven to the lowest heat setting. Line a baking sheet with parchment paper and set aside.

2. Place the cubed potatoes into a small pot, then pour enough cold water to cover them by about an inch. Place over high flame, cover, and bring to a boil. Once boiling, simmer and cook for 8 minutes or until tender.

3. Remove the potatoes from the boiling water with a slotted spoon, then spread them on the prepared baking sheet and place in the oven to keep warm.

4. Meanwhile, blanch the broccoli florets in the boiling water for 1 minute. Drain, then transfer into the oven with the potatoes to keep warm.

5. Pour the lemon juice into a saucepan, then stir in the vinegar, basil, and garlic. Place over medium high flame and bring to a simmer. Once simmering, stir in the parsley, a pinch of red pepper flakes, Dijon mustard, and mustard powder. Stir well, then add the onions and simmer until tender.

6. Stir in the olive oil, then simmer until the dressing is thickened.

7. Transfer the potato and broccoli into a large serving bowl, then pour the hot dressing on top. Toss gently to coat, then serve right away.

Mediterranean Greek Salad

Number of Servings: 3

You will need:

- 1 large head romaine lettuce, torn
- 1 large cucumber, sliced
- 1 large red onion, sliced
- 6 tomatoes, sliced thinly
- 2 Tbsp sliced kalamata olives
- 1 Tbsp crumbled Feta cheese

For the Dressing:

- 1 lemon
- 4 Tbsp extra virgin olive oil
- 1 large garlic clove, crushed
- 1 ½ tsp dried oregano

How to Prepare:

1. Combine the olive oil, garlic, and oregano. Juice and zest the lemon, then whisk into the dressing. Set aside.
2. Toss together the lettuce, cucumber, onion, tomato, and olives in a salad

bowl, then pour the dressing on top and toss well to coat. Add the feta and toss again to combine. Serve right away.

Simple Tomato and Eggplant Stew

Number of Servings: 6

You will need:

- 3 large eggplants, stemmed
- 2 onions, chopped
- 1 large garlic clove, minced
- 3 cups chopped tomatoes, juices reserved
- 3 tsp pure olive oil
- Sea salt, to taste
- Freshly ground black pepper, to taste
- Dried oregano, to taste

How to Prepare:

1. Set the oven to 400 degrees F to preheat.
2. Lay the eggplants on a baking sheet, then drizzle some olive oil on top. Roast for 45 minutes, or until extra tender. Turn once every 15 minutes.
3. Carefully remove the eggplants from the oven and scrape off the flesh. Transfer to a bowl and set aside.

4. Place a large saucepan over medium flame and heat through. Once hot, add the olive oil and swirl to coat. Sauté the onion until tender, then add the garlic and sauté until fragrant.

5. Add the tomatoes and stir until simmering, then add the eggplant and mix well. Simmer until heated through, then season to taste with salt, pepper, and dried oregano.

6. Turn off the heat and allow to cool slightly. Then, puree using an immersion blender or food processor. Reheat over low flame, then serve right away.

Chapter 6 – Seafood, Poultry and Meat Dishes

Moroccan Salmon and Lentils

Number of Servings: 6

You will need:

- 6 large salmon fillets, skin on
- 6 large tomatoes, chopped
- 5 oz green lentils
- 3 large shallots
- 10 garlic cloves
- 2 quarts water
- 4 Tbsp pure olive oil
- 3 Tbsp harissa or other hot sauce
- 1 Tbsp ground fennel seeds
- 1 Tbsp ground coriander
- 1 Tbsp ground cumin
- 1 Tbsp ground cardamom
- ¼ tsp sea salt

- ½ tsp freshly ground black pepper

How to Prepare:

1. Combine the ground spices in a bowl and set aside.

2. Pour the lentils into a saucepan and add the water. Cover and place over high flame, then bring to a boil. Once boiling, reduce to low flame and simmer for 25 minutes or until the lentils are tender, stirring every now and then. Set aside and keep covered.

3. Meanwhile, place a skillet over medium flame and heat through. Add half the olive oil and reduce to low flame. Add the shallots and garlic and let simmer until tender. Add half the spices and stir well to combine. Cook until fragrant.

4. Add the tomatoes with their juices, then simmer until tender. Season to taste with salt and pepper.

5. Set the oven to 350 degrees F to preheat. Blot the salmon with paper towels, then season lightly with salt and pepper. Press the remaining spice mixture all over the salmon.

6. Pour the remaining olive oil over two baking dishes, then swirl to coat. Add the salmon fillets in the baking dishes,

skin side facing down, then bake for 6 to 8 minutes, or until cooked through.

7. Divide the lentils among six plates, then lay a baked salmon on top of each. Ladle the tomato sauce on top, then serve right away.

Italian Poached Fish

Number of Servings: 3

You will need:

- 3 white fish fillets, 4 oz each
- 1 large garlic clove, minced
- ¾ cup chopped tomatoes
- 1/3 cup chopped red onion
- 2 ½ Tbsp dry white wine
- 1 ½ Tbsp capers, rinsed thoroughly
- 1 ½ Tbsp unsalted tomato paste
- 1 ½ Tbsp pure olive oil
- 2 ½ Tbsp chopped fresh parsley

How to Prepare:

1. Place a skillet over medium flame and heat through. Once hot, add the olive oil and swirl to coat. Sauté the onion until translucent, then add the garlic and sauté until fragrant.

2. Stir in the tomato paste, dry white wine, and tomatoes. Bring to a simmer, then stir for 5 minutes.

3. Stir in the capers and mix well. Lay the fish fillets on top and spoon the sauce over the fish to coat. Reduce to low flame, then cover and cook for 10 minutes, or until the fish is completely cooked.

4. Transfer to a serving dish and serve right away.

Mauritian Fish and Herbs

Number of Servings: 6

You will need:

- 3 ¼ lb white fish, such as sea bass or halibut
- 1 large onion, chopped
- 4 garlic cloves, crushed
- 6 large tomatoes, crushed
- 3 Tbsp olive oil
- 3 Tbsp tomato paste
- 2 Tbsp dry sherry
- 2 inches ginger, peeled and crushed
- 2 Tbsp chopped fresh thyme
- 2 Tbsp chopped fresh parsley
- 1 Tbsp chopped fresh coriander
- 1 small lemon, sliced thinly
- Sea salt, to taste
- Freshly ground black pepper, to taste

How to Prepare:

1. Set the oven to 350 degrees F to preheat.
2. Slice the fish into six equal portions, then lay them on a baking dish and season with salt and pepper. Bake for 15 minutes, or until cooked completely.
3. Meanwhile, place a saucepan over medium flame and heat through. Add the oil and swirl to coat. Sauté the onion, garlic, thyme, and ginger until onion is translucent.
4. Stir in the crushed tomatoes and tomato paste, then stir well and bring to a simmer. Cook for 15 minutes.
5. Fold in half the parsley and coriander, then juice the lemon and stir the juice into the mixture. Add the dry sherry and stir well. Bring to a simmer, then season to taste with salt and pepper. Set aside.
6. Once the fish is cooked, carefully remove from the oven and sprinkle the remaining parsley and coriander on top. Set the oven to 400 degrees F.
7. Add the tomato sauce over the fish, then bake again for 10 to 15 minutes, or until the tomato sauce is thickened and bubbly. Best served warm.

Grilled Tuna with Tropical Salsa

Number of Servings: 4

You will need:

- 1 lb tuna steaks, or any other firm fish, sliced into 4 equal pieces
- 1 red bell pepper, seeded and diced
- ½ cup diced pineapple
- ¼ cup diced red onion
- 2 Tbsp chopped fresh cilantro
- 1 Tbsp pure olive oil
- ½ Tbsp white wine vinegar
- Hot pepper sauce, to taste
- Freshly ground black pepper

How to Prepare:

1. Mix together the red onion, pineapple, and bell pepper in a bowl.
2. Fold in the cilantro, then stir in the vinegar. Season to taste with hot sauce, then cover and refrigerate until ready to serve.

3. Preheat the grill to medium flame.
4. Wash the tuna steaks, then blot dry with paper towels. Coat with olive oil, then season all over with black pepper.
5. Grill the tuna steaks for 4 minutes per side, or until cooked through.
6. Lay the tuna steaks on a serving dish, then spoon the tropical salsa on top, then serve right away.

Chicken Cacciatore

Number of Servings: 3

You will need:

- 3 skinless chicken thighs, bone in
- 1 large garlic clove, minced
- 10 oz canned unsalted diced tomatoes, juices reserved
- 1/3 cup chopped onion
- 1/3 cup dry red wine
- 2 ½ Tbsp freshly grated Parmesan cheese
- 1 ½ tsp pure olive oil
- 1 tsp extra virgin olive oil
- ¾ tsp dried parsley
- 1/3 tsp dried oregano
- Freshly ground black pepper, to taste
- 3 cups cooked whole wheat or gluten-free spaghetti, unsalted

How to Prepare:

1. Place a large skillet over medium high flame and heat through. Once hot, add the pure olive oil and swirl to coat. Stir in the onion and sauté until tender.

2. Stir in the garlic, then lay the chicken thighs in a single layer. Cover and cook for 3 minutes per side, or until browned all over.

3. Transfer the chicken thighs to a plate and set aside.

4. Pour in the dry red wine, then add the tomatoes with the juices. Sprinkle in the oregano, parsley, and a pinch of black pepper. Mix well, then increase to high flame and bring to a boil.

5. Once boiling, return the chicken thighs into the pot. Turn to coat, then cover and reduce to medium low flame. Simmer for 10 minutes, then uncover and simmer again for 10 minutes, or until the chicken is cooked through.

6. Divide the pasta among three plates, then lay one chicken thigh on top of each pasta. Ladle the sauce over everything, then drizzle with extra virgin olive oil and serve right away.

Moroccan Honey Chicken and Apricot Tagine

Number of Servings: 6

You will need:

- ❖ 3 large onions, chopped
- ❖ 1 whole chicken, chopped
- ❖ 2 cinnamon sticks
- ❖ 2 cups water
- ❖ 1 cup dried apricots, unsweetened
- ❖ 4 Tbsp grape seed oil
- ❖ 4 Tbsp peeled almonds
- ❖ 3 Tbsp raw honey
- ❖ 1 Tbsp sesame seeds
- ❖ 1 ½ tsp whole black peppercorns
- ❖ ¾ tsp ground turmeric

How to Prepare:

1. Place a saucepan over medium flame and heat through. Once hot, add a bit of the oil and swirl to coat. Sauté the onions until translucent.

2. Add the chopped chicken, then stir in the turmeric, salt, peppercorns, and cinnamon stick. Pour in the water, then bring to a boil.

3. Once boiling, reduce to a simmer, cover, and cook for about 20 minutes or until the chicken is cooked through. Pour in more water, if needed.

4. Transfer the chicken to a serving dish, then cover to keep warm.

5. Add the dried apricots into the saucepan with the sauce. Bring to a boil, then reduce to simmer. Add the honey and simmer, uncovered, until the sauce is thickened. Adjust seasoning to taste. Pour over the chicken and cover again.

6. Place a skillet over medium flame and heat the remaining oil. Add the almonds and stir until golden brown. Transfer the almonds to a plate lined with paper towels and wipe the skillet clean.

7. Reheat the skillet over medium high flame and add the sesame seeds. Stir until toasted, then remove from heat.

8. Sprinkle the almonds and sesame seeds over the chicken dish, then serve right away.

Turkey Florentine

Number of Servings: 3

You will need:

- 3 lean turkey cutlets, 4 oz each
- 4 oz fresh baby spinach
- 1 garlic clove, minced
- ¼ cup dry whole wheat or gluten-free breadcrumbs
- 2 ½ Tbsp shredded Jarlsberg cheese
- 2 Tbsp water
- 1 Tbsp pure olive oil
- 1 Tbsp freshly grated Parmesan cheese
- ¼ tsp ground white pepper
- Ground nutmeg, to taste

How to Prepare:

1. In a deep dish, combine the breadcrumbs, white pepper, and Parmesan cheese. Set aside.

2. Wash the turkey cutlets, then blot dry with paper towels. Place between two sheets of wax paper, then pound as thinly as possible, about an eighth of an inch thick.

3. Moisten the turkey cutlets with the water, shaking off the excess, then dredge them in the breadcrumb mixture. Set aside.

4. Place a saucepan over medium high flame and heat through. Once hot, add the olive oil and reduce to medium flame. Cook the turkey cutlets for 4 minutes per side, or until cooked through.

5. Transfer to a plate lined with paper towels and cover to keep warm.

6. Meanwhile, stir the garlic into the same saucepan. Sauté until fragrant, then stir in the spinach. Add a pinch of nutmeg and stir gently until the spinach is wilted.

7. Sprinkle the Jarlesberg cheese over the spinach, then lay the turkey on top. Cover and turn off the heat.

8. Set aside, covered, for about 3 minutes or until the cheese is melted. Best served warm.

Vegetable and Tender Beef Roast

Number of Servings: 4

You will need:

- 1 ¼ lb bottom round roast, excess fat trimmed off
- 1 small onion, quartered
- 1 large garlic clove, crushed
- 1 large carrot, peeled and cubed
- 2 parsnips, peeled and cubed
- 2 turnips, peeled and chopped
- ½ cup celery, chopped
- 2 medium Yukon Gold potatoes, peeled and quartered
- 2 cups beef broth, unsalted or low sodium
- 2 tsp chili sauce
- ½ Tbsp low sodium soy sauce
- Sea salt, to taste
- Freshly ground black pepper, to taste

How to Prepare:

1. Wash the beef thoroughly, then blot dry with paper towels and season with salt and pepper all over.
2. Place a stock pot over medium high flame and heat through. Once hot, add the beef and cook until browned all over. Transfer to a slow cooker or pressure cooker.
3. Add the onion, garlic, carrot, parsnip, turnip, celery, potatoes, chili sauce, beef broth, and soy sauce in the slow cooker or pressure cooker.
4. Mix well, then cover tightly. If using a slow cooker, cook for 8 hours on low or 4 hours on high. If using a pressure cooker, cook for 50 minutes over medium low flame.
5. Once the beef is tender, carefully transfer it to a large platter and slice thinly. Transfer the sauce and vegetables into a serving bowl, then add the beef on top. Serve right away.

Delhi Lamb and Potatoes

Number of Servings: 4

You will need:

- ¾ lb lamb, diced
- 2 large potatoes, peeled and diced
- 4 large tomatoes, chopped
- 1 large onion, chopped
- 3 garlic cloves, minced
- 7 oz red lentils
- 2 ½ cups water
- 1 ½ Tbsp grape seed oil
- ¾ Tbsp cumin
- 2 tsp sea salt
- ¾ tsp ground coriander
- 1/3 tsp turmeric
- Freshly ground black pepper, to taste
- Cayenne pepper, to taste

How to Prepare:

1. Place a saucepan over medium flame and heat through. Once hot, add the oil and swirl to coat. And swirl to coat. Sauté the onion until tender, then add the garlic and sauté until fragrant.

2. Stir in the diced lamb and sauté for 15 minutes, or until cooked and crumbled. Stir in the cumin, turmeric, coriander, salt, and a pinch of black pepper. Add the tomatoes and stir well. Simmer for 10 minutes, or until sauce is thickened.

3. Add the lentils, potatoes, and water, then bring to a boil. Once boiling, reduce to a simmer and cover. Reduce to the lowest possible heat and simmer for 30 minutes, or until the lentils and potatoes are tender.

4. Uncover and simmer for 10 minutes or until the sauce is thickened. Best served hot.

Grilled Beef and Black Bean Burgers

Number of Servings: 6

You will need:

- 1 lb lean ground beef
- 2 red onions, chopped
- 1 ¼ cups cooked black beans, unsalted
- 1 ½ Tbsp chopped fresh parsley
- 2 fresh cilantro sprigs, chopped
- 1 ¼ tsp ground cumin
- 1 ¼ tsp chili powder
- ½ tsp sea salt

How to Prepare:

1. In a food processor, combine the onion and black beans. Add the cumin, cilantro, parsley, chili powder, cumin, and salt. Blend until smooth.
2. Place the ground beef into a bowl, then fold in the bean mixture. Mix well, hen form into 6 equal sized patties.

3. Lay the patties on a tray and refrigerate for 30 minutes, or until firm and chilled.
4. Meanwhile, preheat the grill to medium flame.
5. Grill the patties for 5 minutes per side, or until cooked through.
6. Transfer to a serving dish and serve with a fresh green salad.

Chapter 7 – Whole Grains

Couscous Curry

Number of Servings: 4

You will need:

- 1 green onion, white and light green parts, chopped
- 1 red onion, diced
- ¾ cup couscous
- ¾ cup boiling water
- ¼ cup diced carrot
- ¼ cup raisins
- ¼ cup minced fresh parsley
- 2 Tbsp slivered almonds
- 2 Tbsp plain non-fat yogurt
- ¾ tsp sesame oil
- ½ Tbsp pure olive oil

- ½ tsp white wine vinegar
- ½ tsp curry powder
- ½ tsp freshly ground black pepper
- 1/8 tsp freshly grated lemon zest
- Turmeric, to taste

How to Prepare:

1. Place the couscous into a heatproof bowl and set aside.
2. Place a skillet over medium flame and heat through. Once hot, add the olive oil and swirl to coat.
3. Stir in the curry powder until fragrant, then add the boiling water and mix well. Pour the mixture over the couscous, then cover the bowl tightly and let stand for 5 minutes.
4. Meanwhile, combine the olive oil, yogurt, lemon zest, and black pepper. Add a pinch of turmeric, then mix well.
5. After 5 minutes, stir the couscous and fluff with a fork. Set aside Pour the yogurt mixture over the couscous and fold well to combine.

6. Add the carrot, raisins, parsley, green onion, red onion, and almonds, then drizzle in the sesame oil and mix well. Serve warm or at room temperature.

Ginger Brown Rice in Avocado

Number of Servings: 6

You will need:

- 3 avocados
- 1 ½ cups uncooked brown rice
- 2 ¼ cups water
- 2 inches fresh ginger, chopped
- 4 ½ Tbsp white wine
- 2 Tbsp raisins
- 2 Tbsp chopped almonds

For the Dressing:

- 1 large lime
- 3 Tbsp extra virgin olive oil
- 1 ½ Tbsp flaxseed oil
- 1 ½ tsp pure maple syrup
- 1 ½ tsp balsamic vinegar
- 1/3 tsp dry mustard
- 1/3 tsp curry powder

How to Prepare:

1. Juice the lime into a bowl, then stir in the olive oil, flaxseed oil, maple syrup, balsamic vinegar, dry mustard, and curry powder. Mix well, then set aside.

2. Combine the water, rice, and ginger in a saucepan, then cover and place over medium high flame. Boil for 15 minutes, then reduce to medium low flame and cook until the rice is tender and has completely absorbed the water.

3. Fold the dressing into the rice, then cover and allow to cool slightly. Transfer to a refrigerator and chill for about 1 hour.

4. Right before serving, halve the avocados and discard the stone, scoop most of the avocado flesh out, then spoon the rice inside. Slice the avocado and lay on top of the rice salad. Serve right away.

Tabbouleh

Number of Servings: 3

You will need:

- 1 large tomato, diced
- 1 garlic clove, minced
- ¾ cup water
- ½ chopped fresh parsley
- ¼ cup bulgur wheat
- ¼ cup chopped green onion
- 2 ½ Tbsp freshly squeezed lemon juice
- 2 Tbsp extra virgin olive oil
- 1 Tbsp chopped fresh mint
- ½ tsp sea salt
- ½ tsp freshly ground black pepper

How to Prepare:

1. Place the bulgur in a bowl, then add the water and mix well. Cover and set aside for 2 hours.

2. After 2 hours, drain the excess water from the bulgur, then transfer to a salad bowl.

3. Fold the chopped garlic, green onion, tomato, parsley, and mint into the bulgur. Add the lemon juice, salt, pepper, and olive oil, then mix well.

4. Cover and refrigerate for 1 to 8 hours, then serve chilled or at room temperature.

Zucchini Whole Wheat Bread

Number of Servings: 10

You will need:

- 1 large egg
- 2 large egg whites
- 1 cup shredded zucchini
- 1 cup whole wheat pastry flour
- ½ cup all-purpose flour
- ½ cup unsweetened applesauce
- 1/3 cup raw honey
- 2 ½ Tbsp canola oil
- 2 ½ Tbsp toasted sunflower seeds
- 1 tsp vanilla paste or extract
- 1 tsp ground cinnamon
- 1 tsp baking powder, low sodium
- ½ tsp sea salt
- ½ tsp baking soda
- ¼ tsp ground nutmeg

- Nonstick cooking spray

How to Prepare:

1. Set the oven to 350 degrees F to preheat. Coat two small aluminum loaf pans with nonstick cooking spray and set aside.
2. In a large bowl, whisk the egg with the egg whites thoroughly. Whisk in the applesauce, honey, canola oil, zucchini, and vanilla paste or extract until thoroughly combined. Set aside.
3. Sift the all-purpose flour and whole wheat flour into another bowl, then mix in the baking soda, baking powder, nutmeg, cinnamon, and salt.
4. Mix the flour mixture into the egg mixture until just combined. Fold in the sunflower seeds.
5. Divide the batter between the two mini loaf pans, then bake for 35 minutes, or until the bread is ready. To check, poke the center of each loaf with a toothpick. If it comes out clean, they loaves are ready.
6. Transfer the loaves onto a cooling rack and allow to cool for 10 minutes. Remove from the pan and allow to cool completely, then slice and serve.

Indonesian Rice Salad

Number of Servings: 4

You will need:

- 2 cups cooked brown rice
- 1 lime or orange
- 1 small garlic clove
- 1 celery stalk, chopped
- 1 green or red bell pepper, seeded and chopped
- 2 spring onions, chopped
- ½ cup crushed pineapple
- 4 ½ Tbsp minced water chestnuts
- 3 Tbsp chopped peanuts
- 3 Tbsp chopped cashews
- 3 Tbsp steamed bean sprouts
- 3 Tbsp raisins
- 3 Tbsp peanut oil
- 2 Tbsp sesame oil
- 1 ½ Tbsp sesame seeds

- 1 ½ Tbsp low sodium soy sauce
- 1 ½ Tbsp apple cider vinegar
- ¾ tsp sea salt
- Cayenne pepper, to taste

How to Prepare:

1. Place the cooked brown rice into a serving bowl, then fold in the sesame and peanut oils. Juice the lime or orange, then fold the juice into the rice.
2. Season with garlic, salt, soy sauce, vinegar, and cayenne pepper to taste. Fold in the pineapple, water chestnut, celery, spring onion, bean sprouts, peanuts, cashews, raisins, sesame seeds, and bell pepper.
3. Cover the bowl and refrigerate for at least an hour. Best served chilled.

Oatmeal, Banana and Raspberry Loaf

Number of Servings: 6

You will need:

- 1 ripe banana, peeled and mashed
- 1 large egg white
- 1 egg
- 1 ½ oz low fat cream cheese, softened
- ½ cup all-purpose flour
- ½ cup fresh raspberries
- ¼ cup traditional rolled oats
- ¼ cup whole wheat flour
- 3 Tbsp blackstrap molasses
- 2 Tbsp freshly squeezed orange juice
- ½ tsp baking soda
- ½ tsp baking powder

How to Prepare:

1. Set the oven to 350 degrees F to preheat.
2. Combine the blackstrap molasses with the cream cheese in a bowl, then beat until fluffy. Add the mashed banana, orange juice, egg white, and egg. Mix well until smooth.
3. Sift together the whole wheat flour, all-purpose flour, baking soda, and baking powder. Fold the flour into the egg mixture until just combined. Add the oats and raspberries, then mix well.
4. Pack the batter into a nonstick loaf pan and bake for 35 to 40 minutes, or until golden brown.
5. To check, poke the center of each loaf with a toothpick. If it comes out clean, they loaves are ready.
6. Transfer the loaves onto a cooling rack and allow to cool for 10 minutes. Remove from the pan and allow to cool completely, then slice and serve.

Chapter 8 – Desserts

Honey Cinnamon Fruit Medley

Number of Servings: 8

You will need:

- 1 small cantaloupe
- 3 apples
- 3 bananas
- 5 oranges, peeled, seeded, and sliced
- 2 lemons
- 3 Tbsp raw honey
- 1 ½ tsp pure vanilla extract
- 1 ½ tsp ground cinnamon

How to Prepare:

1. Combine the honey, vanilla extract, and cinnamon in a bowl. Juice one lemon, then stir the juice into the honey mixture and set aside.

2. Halve the cantaloupe and scoop out the flesh with a melon baller or slice into bite sized cubes. Place in a large bowl.

3. Peel and slice the bananas, then add to the fruit bowl. Add the sliced oranges.

4. Core and cube the apples, then place in a small bowl. Juice the other lemon over it and toss well to coat. Pour everything into the fruit bowl.

5. Pour the honey cinnamon mixture over the fruit mixture, then toss well to coat. Refrigerate for at least 1 hour before serving. Best served chilled.

Carrot Lemon Cake

Number of Servings: 12

You will need:

- 6 large eggs, separated
- 2 ¼ cups freshly grated carrot
- ¾ cup brown sugar
- ¾ cup whole wheat flour
- 4 ½ Tbsp freshly grated lemon zest
- 1 ½ Tbsp freshly squeezed lemon juice
- 2 ¼ tsp baking soda
- ¾ tsp sea salt
- 1 ½ inches fresh ginger, peeled and minced
- Nonstick cooking spray

How to Prepare:

1. Set the oven to 325 degrees F to preheat. Lightly coat a large baking pan with nonstick cooking spray and set aside.

2. In a bowl, beat the egg whites with an electric mixer until soft peaks. Set aside.

3. In a separate bowl, beat together the grated carrot, egg yolks, and sugar. Mix in the lemon zest, lemon juice, and whole wheat flour until smooth. Next, beat in the baking soda, salt, and ginger.

4. Fold the egg whites into the batter, then pour the batter into the baking pan.

5. Bake for 1 hour, or until golden brown. To check, poke the center of the cake with a toothpick. If it comes out clean, they cake is ready.

6. Transfer the cake onto a cooling rack and allow to cool for 10 minutes. Remove from the pan and allow to cool completely, then slice and serve.

No-Bake Almond Pumpkin Spice Bites

Number of Pieces: 30

You will need:

- 1 ½ lb dark chocolate chips
- 1 ¼ cups almond butter
- ¾ cup pureed pumpkin
- 1 ¼ tsp raw honey
- ¾ tsp ground cinnamon
- 1/3 tsp ground cardamom
- 1/3 tsp ground ginger
- 1/3 tsp allspice

How to Prepare:

1. Line muffin tins with paper liners, then set aside.
2. Melt half the chocolate chips in the microwave or double boiler. Pour the melted chocolate into the prepared muffin tins, coating the bottom evenly. Refrigerate for later.

3. Combine the almond butter, pureed pumpkin, honey, cinnamon, cardamom, ginger, and allspice in a food processor. Blend until smooth.

4. Remove the muffin tins from the refrigerator, then divide the pumpkin mixture among them. Divide the remaining chocolate chips on top, then refrigerate for at least 1 hour, or until set. Best served chilled.

Baked Oatmeal-Stuffed Apples

Number of Servings: 6

You will need:

- 3 large apples, cored and halved
- 3 Tbsp water
- 6 tsp brown sugar
- 4 tsp traditional rolled oats
- 2 tsp hot water
- 3 tsp freshly squeezed lemon juice
- Ground cinnamon, to taste
- Nonstick cooking spray

How to Prepare:

1. Set the oven to 375 degrees F to preheat. Lightly coat a baking dish with nonstick cooking spray.
2. Lay the cut apples on the prepared baking dish, sliced side facing up. Sprinkle the lemon juice on top to prevent browning. Set aside.
3. In a bowl, combine the rolled oats and hot water until pasty. Add the brown sugar, then mix well. Spoon the mixture

on top of the halved apples, then coat the apples lightly with nonstick cooking spray.

4. Sprinkle the ground cinnamon on top of the apples, then pour the water around them into the pan.
5. Bake for 30 minutes, or until the apples are hot and fork tender. Serve warm or chilled.

Nutty Chocolate Chip Cookies

Number of Servings: 12

You will need:

- 1 ½ cups chopped walnuts
- 9 Medjool dates, pitted and chopped
- ¾ cup unsweetened applesauce
- ¾ cup flaxseed meal
- ½ cup dark chocolate chips
- 1/3 cup unsweetened coconut flakes
- 1/3 cup almond butter
- 1 ½ tsp vanilla extract
- ¾ tsp baking soda
- Sea salt, to taste

How to Prepare:

1. Set the oven to 350 degrees F to preheat. Line a baking sheet with parchment paper and set aside.

2. Place the dates and walnuts into a food processor and blend until chunky. Pour in the almond butter, applesauce, vanilla extract, and a pinch of salt. Blend until smooth with bits of walnut.

3. Combine the coconut flakes, baking soda and flaxseed meal. Add the walnut mixture and fold well until thoroughly combined. Fold in the chocolate chips.

4. Scoop the dough into small balls, about 2 inches in diameter each. Flatten with a fork, then bake for 10 minutes.

5. Turn the cookies over, then bake for an additional 5 minutes, or until firm but still gooey.

6. Transfer to a cooling rack and allow to cool completely. Place in an airtight cooking jar.

Lemon Pear Cream

Number of Servings: 3

You will need:

- ¾ oz pasteurized egg white
- 1/6 oz unflavored gelatin
- ¾ cup pear nectar
- ¾ cup non-fat lemon yogurt
- ¼ cup freshly squeezed lemon juice
- 2 ½ Tbsp cold water
- ¾ tsp freshly grated lemon zest
- 1/6 tsp cream of tartar

How to Prepare:

1. Mix together the gelatin and cold water in a microwaveable glass bowl. Set aside for 5 minutes.
2. After 5 minutes, add the lemon juice and pear nectar. Mix well, then microwave for 1 minute and 30 seconds on high, stirring once every 30 seconds.

3. Carefully remove from the microwave, then stir in the lemon zest. Set aside and allow to cool to room temperature.

4. Meanwhile, beat the egg whites with the cream of tartar until soft peaks start to form.

5. Once the gelatin mixture is cooled, stir in the lemon yogurt. Fold in the egg white mixture, then divide among three parfait glasses. Refrigerate for at least 4 hours, or until chilled. Best served chilled.

Conclusion

Hopefully this book has helped you treat or prevent your thyroid condition and achieve your overall health goals. Maximize the benefits of this book by creating a meal plan that will encourage you to continue preparing and eating nutritious home-cooked meals.

Stay motivated and inspired to take good care of your body, because if you really stop to think about it, it is your most valuable asset. So eat right and be healthy!

Made in the USA
San Bernardino, CA
12 November 2016